Nation Heal Thyself

A Primary Prevention Guide:
Comprehensive and Holistic,
Functional, and Includes a One and
Only Prevention Healthscore

by
Dr. Malik H. Dababneh

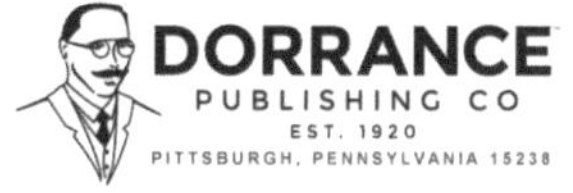

Dorrance Publishing Co
585 Alpha Drive
Pittsburgh, PA 15238
Visit our website at www.dorrancebookstore.com

ISBN: 979-8-8860-4131-6
eISBN: 979-8-8860-4796-7

Twenty-seven years in medicine

Ten years in federal custody

Four years in federal prison

Seven years of combined outpatient and inpatient treatment for marijuana addiction

The Doctor Pusher

The Future of Family Medicine report, released in 2004, concluded that the US healthcare system was inadequate and unsustainable, and that without transformation, the specialty of family medicine might be in danger of extinction. From this call to action, a host of innovation and projects were born. These include the Annals of Family Medicine, launched with the goal of improving and expanding primary care-focused research. The Preparing the Personal Physician for Practice (P4) Initiative for innovation in family medicine residency education was launched in 2007 and continues to be mined for lessons on graduate medical education redesign. Family Medicine for America's Health and Health is Primary initiatives followed in 2012 and 2014 with particular focus on the triple aim of improving population health, experience of care, and per capita coast, as well as positioning family medicine as an essential player in the changing healthcare climate.

After nearly 2 decades, family medicine has achieved many of the initial aims of the Future of Family Medicine report and has helped shape national health policy. Yet the fact remains that healthcare in the United States remains inadequate and unsustainable. It is unsustainable financially in that more than 90% of the $3.8 trillion in healthcare expenditures is spent on chronic disease and mental health conditions. Healthcare costs grow faster than inflation, and individuals and corporations alike struggle under the financial burden of obtaining healthcare. One example: An explosion of new medications for diabetes has revolutionized the national guidelines, yet the diabetes epidemic grows unabated. Despite all the innovations in healthcare

Supplement The Journal of Family Practice. Vol. 71 No. 1. Jan/Feb 2022. Page 566-569. Author Brenda Rea MD Dr PH PT RD, Philip Johnson MD, et al. ? doi 10.12788/Jfp.0273

design, delivery, technology, patient-centered efforts, medical home initiatives, and data analysis, as well as pharmacologic advances, we have failed to advance in our efforts to help individuals and society at large with the foundational elements that support healthy lifestyle behaviors.

The culmination of this, part memoir part health care guide, is an eighteen-year effort that began with a traffic ticket in Michigan and ended in Federal prison. The aim has always been to teach and empower my patients to use their God given, uniquely human qualities to better themselves and help others. In my three decades of practice, the art of medicine has moved from a patriarchal system, where medical advice is handed down in a fatherly fashion, to a more sophisticated and evidence-based healthcare delivery. It is necessary to partner with our patients to improve access, control costs, raise quality of life, and extend longevity. Recent times of social unrest and a viral pandemic that hasn't been felt since the Spanish flu over a hundred years ago mandates an evolutionary change. It has been well-established for many years that prevention of disease is the key. Doctors have come a long ways in treating illness by using the bio psychosocial model to assess and diagnose individuals. Doctor-patient interactions are usually intense and can bring about negative feelings, and that's why I created this guide and the SPOKE WHEEL HOLISTIC HEALTHSCORE. This is a self-assessment score based on twenty questions, that includes all the health parameters. This is a tangible tool that is easy to use. I've practiced both traditional and holistic medicine in small towns and large cities and in urgent care centers and emergency rooms. I can tell you that 80 percent of disease or injury is preventable. I use the bio psychosocial spiritual model to heal and prevent illness. Prevention of disease is the key to health, happiness, and longevity. Gaining balance in certain areas of life while navigating medical complexities is the crux of this guide.

While in prison, someone handed me an article clipping from the Detroit News that listed me as one of Michigan's doctor drug pushers. A drug pusher is like a corner street drug dealer that sells drugs to teenagers. I was embarrassed, angry, and humiliated. I had already been imprisoned for a couple of years, trying to accept my culpability in this conspiracy, while coming to terms with surrendering my freedom and career and abandoning my family. What hurt the most was the unnecessary and traumatizing ransacking of my home by armed federal agents, while being handcuffed and rifles pointed at me and my wife. My daughter was forced to lay prone while another agent pointed a gun at her. The search warrant yielded nothing. No guns, no drugs, no money, and no evidence of wrongdoing. This was nothing compared to the guilt I felt and the anger that followed when my younger brother, Majed, developed heart disease and died, and I was denied a furlough to be with him. In my years of practice, I did everything I could to help my patients. In fact I spent countless hours counseling people to come off drugs or reduce their intake and find healthy ways to control their pain. This is a timely guide to stay healthy and live longer. Find out how to eliminate anxiety and stress within minutes. Get the nuts, the bolts, and the tools to fix what ails you.

The first time I heard the phrase, "...heal thyself, " I was a confused and excitable teenage boy who just became fluent in English as a second language. I and a group of neighborhood friends were invited to the local Springwells Baptist church where I became a born-again Christian. I grew up Catholic, in the mostly Muslim Middle East, and was baptized in the River Jordan as an infant. My family and I immigrated to Detroit, Michigan in 1967 when I was eight and the eldest of three siblings. We had been displaced from Jericho and further impoverished by war between Israel and Egypt, only to arrive in Detroit during the race riots.

At the time, I didn't know that I would become a successful doctor, only to eventually fall from grace and hit a rock bottom that would derail my career after decades of hard work. It would be some fifty years later that I would hear that phrase again sitting in a federal prison. Saint Luke, who wrote one of the four gospels, was believed to be a physician.

In Luke 4:23, "cura te ipsum," which in Latin means *physician heal thyself*. This was a quoted proverb of Jesus when questioned about political and societal ills that were present in Ancient Rome. A similar quote of Jesus in Mathew 9:9-13 when referring to miracles and individual health. After years of trying to help others, I was finally forced to work on myself.

In prison I thought about my childhood, my family, and my patients. I wanted to put on paper what I had been afraid to do for myself because I felt trapped in a cycle that was spinning out of control. I needed to stop spinning and reassess my situation and try to practice what I had been teaching my patients. I wanted to tell people ways they could improve their health. By putting it on paper, it also helped reinforce it in my own head.

I recall, by age twelve, I had developed so much anger that I unleashed it on a sixteen-year-old bully and almost killed him. It was a hot summer day, and my friend and I were walking to the corner grocery store where I had a part-time job. The kid was named Piggy and was part of a street gang that patrolled the corner, and that day he was alone and demanded money from me as an entrance fee to the store. The next thing I remember is kicking him in the groin with my knee and then I broke his nose with a vicious upper cut. I proceeded to pound his head into the wall and the concrete sidewalk while straddling his chest.

Thank God that I was brought to my sense by his eighteen-year-old sister, who was bigger than both of us and had witnessed what was happening. She tackled me with a leap from her porch across the street with the expertise of an NFL linebacker. At the time of the incident, I felt a rush and a relief of my anger, but later it turned into guilt and then anxiety.

I had periods of anxiety after because I lived in Southwest Detroit where there had been a lot of gang violence, and I remember that there were times I was walking home in the dark and would walk through a dangerous ally on purpose to confront my fears.

Immaturity

As young teens growing up in Detroit and being people of color, my brother Majed and I were bullied by gangs and physically assaulted. We were forced to defend ourselves at a very young age. I remember that starting around age nine getting beat up and regularly being teased and called camel or sand nigger. At thirteen I was robbed of my newspaper route money at knifepoint by a gang of three young men (two Black and one Mexican). When I was seventeen and my brother Majed was fifteen, we were assaulted by a motorcycle gang because the color of our skin (they were white). I somehow managed to talk our way out of a potentially dangerous encounter, Against all odds, we avoided dealing in drugs and criminal life. Unlike many of my high school friends who ended up in jail or dead either selling heroin or overdosing, I was fortunate because I had a loving and supportive family

By the time I was fifteen, I was thrust into adulthood. I knew I had to work hard to get out of the city and escape violence and poverty. I became the hero child. I remember having two part-time jobs and doing well in school, as well as playing sports, doing theater, and participating in art exhibits at my high school. I was the eldest boy of a large immigrant family of color in an increasingly racist and divided society and felt the extra pressure to succeed.

When I began using marijuana at fifteen, it relieved the emotional pain, childhood oppression, and depression that I had growing up. It allowed me to deal with the aggression that I abhorred and to deal with the trauma and sexual abuse that occurred at the hands of a neighborhood couple. I was seduced by the couple and encouraged by the husband to have sex with his wife. I was twelve when I had sex for the first time, and it felt good. I also felt guilt and shame. I didn't know what that was at the time. I felt extremely sad, and I knew what that was and did not like it. I was from a culture that did not believe in premarital sex and yet I had sex with a married woman, and it made me feel great and yet like an adulterer, which for me was a sin. I don't have a good recollection of what happened that summer, but I did have sex with her several times. It all came to a stop when her husband tried to have oral sex with me. For some reason that was a line I refused to cross, however something eventually clicked that summer and at that moment I began to work on my American dream, maybe this was the moment I was forced into adulthood. They stole my innocence and morally corrupted me for years to come. I felt my hope crushed and my spiritual maturity stalled. Years of suppressed feelings and fears that were dominated by shame and guilt resulted in decades of back-breaking work. I used all that emotional energy to fuel my desire to succeed. I put aside my depression and became obsessed with success. I would bury the deep sadness I felt of being exposed to war and senseless killing that forced me out of my own country just several years prior. I hid the memory of seeing dead bodies and slit throats and chest and head wounds and airplanes dropping bombs. But deep down inside, I wanted to understand it or even try to fix it. I was already feeling depressed upon arriving to this country, yet I was elated to leave war and famine. I was overjoyed to be with family, but the culture shock was almost too much for a young dark Arab boy who did not speak English. So I learned English, worked hard, excelled, and luckily became a doctor. Perhaps this is why I ultimately chose medicine as a profession. I could gain wealth and notoriety and really make a difference.

For years I had been teaching my patients to create balance in their lives and to combat illness, and how imbalance in our lives affects our mental and physical well-being. But the problem was that I wasn't totally practicing what I was preaching, and my own life was spinning out of control. After I graduated from Michigan State university, college of osteopathic medicine, I was responsible for opening outreach clinics for the Indian health service in northern Michigan. I served on staff at the local hospitals and worked some of the emergency rooms in northern Michigan and the upper peninsula. I enjoyed doing house calls because it gave me a glimpse of how people live and how it affects their health. I completed my work with the Indian health service after almost five years in exchange for three years of tuition. In the early nineties, I moved and worked in rural Illinois where I delivered babies, performed circumcisions, and took care of my own emergency room patients and ICU patients. I was medical director of several nursing homes and was president of the Fulton County medical society in Illinois. I had been appointed adjunct clinical instructor at MSU in Michigan and Midwestern in Illinois. By the time I moved back to Michigan, I felt overworked and overwhelmed. 9/11 just happened, and that didn't help matters. I was a middle-aged, dark-skinned Arab doctor who was just too busy or afraid to stop, take a deep breath, and look into the mirror.

Maturing

Landing in prison was both a curse and a blessing. I abandoned my family and patients. I surrendered my medical license and lost my freedom. Truly there were times that I wanted to go to trial because my case arose out of civil negligence and not conspiracy to distribute narcotics, which in the eyes of the law is the same as a street corner drug dealer. In 2011 I was indicted on charges of Medicare fraud and conspiracy to distribute narcotics. I was told by the federal prosecutor that the FBI and DEA had been following me since 2009. One reason, potentially, is I had a possession of marijuana misdemeanor on my record from 2003. Ironically it was because of my criminal record that I was working for multiple pain clinics in Detroit, and in 2010 I was hired by a home health clinic owner to supervise physician assistants doing home visits. This turned out to be a fraudulent operation as the owner and operator eventually became a federal witness (aka confidential informant) in exchange to reduce charges. Three separate law firms told me my chances of winning were slim to none because the prosecutor held all the cards, and the chances of winning were less than 5 percent. In fact the judge was likely to give me more time for proceeding with trial because if found guilty, he could add additional time for "obstruction of justice." The judge, the prosecutors, and usually the defense team work together to save time and money for the federal government. Even defense attorneys generally don't want to create future problems for the court and are oftentimes agreeable with the prosecution or don't want the headache of going to trial.

Moreover the country was in the midst of an opioid epidemic, and unprecedented overdoses were occurring across the heartland. Medicare fraud was also on the rise, and the department of justice was under pressure to solve this problem. Many health professionals became targets and even willing and unwilling scapegoats. The feds and the marketers were using unscrupulous methods to get their way. Many legal and medical scholars and professionals would agree that we have a failed criminal justice system. We continue to have a high recidivism rate despite the many rehabilitation programs. One reason for this failure is that federal laws make it almost impossible for many felons to re-enter society. We are forced to surrender our professional licenses and passports. Felons are denied certain rights, including voting and other commerce related opportunities like traveling and working or partnering with family. There are many obstacles in place that prevent true rehabilitation and reform. In reality my case should have been settled in civil court, but instead I was indicted on federal conspiracy charges, along with 100 other defendants, most of whom I've never had contact nor association. The prosecutors across the country were under pressure to get convictions, and doctors became perfect rallying points and targets, especially those that were providing a much-needed service of working in those needy areas. I've certainly never had the intention to conspire or distribute drugs illegally.

What's more is the complicated relationship between the Federal bureau of prisons and the department of justice and how the judicial system creates the "prison industrial complex." One feature of this is that federal prisoners are bonded on a stock exchange system on Wall Street, and that currency is available to federal judges and prosecutors and some senators. I can only confirm this as a rumor passed by well-informed inmates some who had been states congressman, attorneys, and other professionals who are knowledgeable with corporate and Wall Street dealings. In this country, there are small towns where the largest employer is the federal bureau of prisons, and all their subsidiary contractors actually employ half the town. The United States and Philippines are the only countries that have a cash-based bond system for qualified individuals. This creates a disparity in justice based on wealth and bias.

My incarceration included plenty of long-needed rest. I had plenty of time to think and write and draw and try to reach out and make amends the best I could. I was very lucky to have the support of my family, especially my wife and children. In prison I also taught other inmates art, GED classes, senior care business classes, health and nutrition classes, and although I couldn't practice nor give medical advice, nor even being referred to as a doctor, sometimes inmates and guards sought my medical advice. For example one guard asked me to see another inmate who was having stroke symptoms in the middle of the night while awaiting staff help. At another time and a different inmate and guard it was chest pain. One night I had to get a random drug test, and while waiting to give my urine, actually advised the guard how he could give up tobacco. He had switched to chewing to avoid smoking while at work and inadvertently doubled his nicotine use. We talked about balance, and who knows what happened after that. This is not to mention the inmates with their personal struggles with addiction, mental health, pain issues, family issues, including dealing with cancer. I felt a sense of pride but also resentment. I had to let go of blaming my past and forgive myself and others and learn to accept my present circumstances.

It took years for me to finally accept some responsibility for my actions and years of therapy and self-analysis to realize what was mentally torturing me and how it led me astray.

For years I believed that I could achieve any goal as long as I worked hard and treated others as I would want to be treated. This philosophy was working well for me, but I was neglecting some very important things that were going on around me. I had moved back to Michigan after 9/11, and one year later, my father died. He was the reason I moved back. I was doing very well in Illinois but wanted to be closer to him.

Things changed when my father died. He was my rock and anchor. The person who always managed to make me feel good was suddenly gone. Back during the war, my father was almost shot by an Israeli soldier as we were cutting through the orchard to get to the church basement for a bomb shelter. I only had bits and pieces of that memory, but my father often retold and that the soldier did not shoot because he was wearing a cross. I was feeling especially bad in prison; one day I received a thoughtful letter from one of my daughters that said that I was the one who taught her how to laugh. It brought me to tears, and that's when I realized what my own father had meant to me. After my father passed, I spent the next ten years in a deep cycle of guilt and blame that led to debilitating self-pity and inconsolable grief. I was smoking marijuana regularly, and by the time the federal government caught up with me, I was fifty-five and on the verge of financial ruin. I made many wrong choices, mostly because I was not willing to let go and forgive myself. I was busy caring for others and neglecting my own mental and physical and even spiritual health. I was ignoring warning signs and hitting bumps in the road and did not stop nor even slow down to balance the spokes on my wheel. I was even neglecting my medical licensure. When hardship began for me, I blamed others, and it took years for me to begin taking some responsibility for my choices and actions.

Because of what I can only describe as a comedy of errors within the bureaucracy of the federal system of prisons, and my own naivety, I was not given my long-standing blood pressure medication for the first few months, which put me at great risk of a stroke or a heart attack. I knew the dangers of this, and as a doctor, I had to take orders from a physician assistant who did not like me, nor did he care whether I lived or died. He had full control of the direction of my healthcare. This scared the hell out me, and I felt very vulnerable. In fact my blood pressure spiked to 180/120, which is stroke-level dangerous.

I began to understand what a patient would feel like to be left helpless at the hands of healthcare providers. It is similar to helplessness at the hand of large organizations, like insurance companies or Medicare and Medicaid and the Veterans Administration. Over the years, I met and took care of a lot of people with no insurance and gave free care like many doctors do.

Professional courtesy is nice, but one of the greatest gifts a doctor can give his patient is to empower him or her with the medical knowledge that would result in the most favorable outcome. This only comes from experience, wisdom, and knowing your patients.

We need a healthcare and disease prevention system that goes beyond the bio-psychosocial model and where logic, common sense, and an understanding of culture and human nature are used in keeping the body in homeostasis. I call it the bio-psychosocio-spiritual model.

Matured

I created a spoke wheel to best describe what is needed to keep in balance and how. The wheel represents the body, and the road is life. It has eight spokes that represent major areas that are necessary to keep in balance. Each spoke has four prongs attached to the rim and center hub, which is your inner self and/or higher power. The rim and tire represent your condition and genetic makeup. Basically the shape you are currently in.

You will less likely drift off the path of a road if your tires are in good shape and each spoke is tightly balanced. Use the prongs to tighten each spoke. This will be discussed later.

One of my proudest moments and best compliments that I often think about was when one of my many patients told me that I restored his faith in doctors. He said I saved his life because I diagnosed kidney cancer in him with his only symptom or worry was persistently borderline elevated blood pressure. Almost all medical professionals will tell you that a diagnosis can be made by taking a careful history of the patient 80 percent of the time. That means listening to your patients.

I reflect on that because many people have lost their faith in the healthcare system. Long before there was Medicaid and Medicare, large hospitals corporations and universities, the physician, your general practitioner spent unhurried hours taking care of your family for whatever you could afford to pay him, sometimes in exchange for eggs or a chicken. Even today many doctors and providers serve their community with that same caring ethos and passion.

A recent study conducted by the American Academy of Family Physicians in 2016 concluded, "the current medical school system is failing, collectively, to produce the primary care work force that is needed to achieve optimal health" (Fam Med. 2016; 48[9]:688-95). This tells me that medical schools are misguided and focus more on economics rather than individual health and produce doctors that focus on treatment rather than prevention. I know because I was a product of that system. The United States has the best medical schools in the world and is the richest and most powerful nation, and yet we have had devastating COVID-19 deaths and continue to struggle to provide the best care for our citizens on an equitable and fair scale.

Prior to release, I spent the last few months of incarceration in quarantine isolation as a precaution and then released to home confinement during a nationwide "pandemic lockdown." When I left prison, there were 60,000 COVID deaths, and one year later, there are more than half a million deaths, twice the rate predicted.

Part of the initial treatment for COVID-19 is vitamin C, that I have recommended for twenty-five years. Vitamin C has been controversial for many years because it lacks medical evidence in its efficacy to fight infection. Omega 3 fish oil recently gained acceptance for its cardiac benefits (but not yet for joint or brain health), but I could not get it during my time with the feds because it was not FDA approved. Indeed I have been advocating vitamin C and Omega 3, as well as other things outlined in my medical pearls of wisdom, for my patients, family, and myself for decades. In the following pages, I will outline a holistic disease prevention and health guide, where I will ask you to take a self-assessment questionnaire, and then I will discuss a balanced approach to wellness. The FDA does what it can to regulate the onslaught of drugs entering the market, but it can be influenced by money as we have seen in the ongoing investigation of this opioid epidemic. Purdue pharmaceutical was given special reduced addictive potential status for its drug, OxyContin, which eventually influenced doctors decisions to prescribe it. When the person can no longer get the drug from the doctor, they often turn to the streets to get drugs. Ironically, but not surprisingly, one of the FDA commissioners later became a board member for Purdue pharmaceutical. When a doctor prescribes OxyContin for pain, and the patient becomes addicted and can no longer get the prescription legally, they often turn to heroin or alcohol to satisfy their emotional and physical pain.

Consider this guide a set of tools that you and your health provider can use to identify areas of concern and then attempt to specifically target what can be corrected or improved upon. It is intended for you to take an honest self-appraisal of your entire life from the perspective of total wellness. There are no right or wrong answers, but to make it easier to follow, I created twenty important questions to rate each from one to five for a total of 100 points, which is the best score. The lowest score is twenty. Having said that, I scored seventy-three the first time I took it, and I was being generous to myself.

Obviously the objective would be to score better the next time you do the self-assessment. That could be one month or one year depending on your health needs; for example, if you have hypertension and you are a smoker, you might take the test a couple times a year. If you have severe anxiety, you could try to manage the test daily. If you struggle with anxiety, read on.

Medicine for me is fascinating, especially when you consider that a human organism is made of tens of trillions of cells that function individually, yet communicate with the rest of the body and mind to make a person whole. How our minds can choose to live in the past, present, and future or all three at once amazes me. Twins who have been separated at birth and never met will have interconnected feelings for each other. The enigma of medicine is that a serious condition can seem benign and vice versa while some disease will create different symptoms in differing patients.

About twenty years ago, while working on a Native American reservation in northern Michigan, a patient came to see me for chest pain. He was a diabetic, obese smoker, and I spent considerable time educating him from a holistic standpoint, which it seemed to have a noticeable effect on him. Within a short time, he made tremendous strides in improving his health and social outcome. His chest pain was caused by anxiety. A careful examination revealed that he had imbalances in his spoke wheel, specifically his physical and mental health, as well as relationships issues with his wife and daughter.

I also took care of a middle-age woman who came to me for persistent leg pain. She had no insurance and avoided seeing a doctor for months.

I took an X-ray and diagnosed metastatic bone cancer because of a well-established apple core lesion; an apple core lesion is an X-ray finding where the bone looks like it had a "bite" taken out of it that was typical in bone cancer. She died six months later. I gave her palliative care at home and was there when she passed.

I have literally taken care of tens of thousands of patients over my career, and I'm not sure why it seems that certain individuals keep popping back in my mind, but these are some of the people I think about when I write this guide. This woman was standing out in my mind for a number of reasons but primarily because of the delicate relationship between her and her younger sisters. She was ready to go, but they were unwilling to let go of her. Her pain was excruciating because it was bone pain. I placed her on a morphine drip to control it, and we prayed aloud and silently. Peace eventually found her.

Prevention

The man I admire most is Jesus Christ because he was a carpenter, teacher, and healer who died as he had lived. He gave us the golden rule, ``which is to love thy neighbor and treat others as you would want to be treated. He showed how one must live by the ultimate example of acceptance and forgiveness.

A quote from the great philosopher, Frederick Nietzche, "Christ legacy to mankind: His behavior before his accusers and his judges and on the cross where he does not resist nor defend his right. He begs, suffers, and loves those who do evil to him. He is not angry and does not hold the evil one responsible, on the contrary, He loves him."

Growing up in Jordan and at a young age, I knew that I wanted to live right. I was an altar boy at a Catholic church, and I learned early on to fear the seven deadly sins. Ancient wisdom from many religions teach us to avoid gluttony, envy, lust, wrath, pride, agreed, and sloth, for they will surely lead to misery and decline.

In psychology we talk about the positive attitudes that we use to right any wrongs and to make amends with the world and try to live the best possible life that you can live; these are responsibility, honesty, caring, open-mindedness, objectivity, willingness, humility, and gratitude, as well as empathy and selflessness.

Aristotle, around 350 B.C., was the first physician to document that we humans have a combination of physical and spiritual properties, and there is no separation between mind and body. Medicine is in a state of transition, and we as a nation could be better prepared to prevent another viral pandemic We would be better prepared to handle a pandemic by following certain guidelines and possibly having comprehensive national healthcare.

In this guide, I use ancient and modern medicine to get a better understanding of our health and how we can use balance to create wellness, longevity, through disease prevention.

Hippocrates, a Greek physician who lived almost 500 years before Christ, also known as the father of medicine, is quoted as saying that illness does not come out of the blue, they are developed from small daily sins of nature, and when enough sins have accumulated, illness will suddenly appear. We can prevent obesity, diabetes, hypertension, infection, injuries, mental illness, and some cancers.

It is said that an ounce of prevention is worth a pound in cure. Most doctors don't discuss prevention because they are too busy treating disease. Prevention of primary disease is the aim of this guide. Primary disease, like obesity, hypertension, diabetes, depression and anxiety, addiction, and infection, are preventable. If left untreated they will lead to disability, illness, and premature death. Although trauma is not considered a disease per se, it is preventable in most cases and plays a major role in disability and chronic pain and rising health care costs.

The following few pages have a list of questions that will be used to assess our health and wellness. This will be followed by the spoke wheel holistic guide.

HEALTHSCORE ASSESSMENT
Health Assessment Questionnaire

- **Weight** - (BMI = Body Mass Index)
    5= normal
    4= mild obesity
    3= moderate obesity
    2= morbid obesity
    1= morbid obesity after bypass surgery

- **Blood pressure**
    5= normal or controlled with medication
    4= uncontrolled with medication
    3= uncontrolled and non-compliant
    2= uncontrolled with symptoms of disease
    1= uncontrolled with heart disease

- **Diabetes**
    5= none or glycohemoglobin A1C less 5 no meds
    4= normal sugars or glycohemoglobin A1C between 5 and 6.4
        with medical therapy
    3= glycohemoglobin A1C between 6.5 and 8.5 with medical therapy
    2= glycohemoglobin A1C above 8.5 with therapy
    1= glycohemoglobin A1C above 8.5 and non-compliant

- **Lipids/cholesterol**
  5= normal
  4= borderline or diet controlled
  3= elevated
  2= elevated with maximum medical therapy
  1= elevated with known heart disease

- **Cardiac/stroke/ blood clot/aneurysm**
  5= no history or very low risk
  4= low risk
  3= moderate risk
  2= high risk (example, obese diabetic smoker that is non-compliant with therapy)
  1= current ongoing disease like a recent heart attack or stroke

- **Sleep**
  5= normal
  4= less than five hours of continuous sleep
  3= require sleep medication several times monthly including alcohol or marijuana
  2= require routine use of meds or substance to stay asleep or fall asleep
  1= difficulty sleeping no matter what
  (basically, Michael Jackson syndrome)

- **Exercise**
  5= forty five minutes or more daily
  4= fifteen to twenty minutes daily
  3= exercise once or twice per week or weekends only
  2= rarely exercise
  1= never exercise

■ Meditation/Prayer

5= daily practice sixty minutes or more of some form of spiritual
exercise

4= twenty minutes or more

3= weekly practice

2= rarely

1= never

■ Anger/Resentment

5= occasional and temporary

4= anger and resentment toward enemies

3= anger and resentment towards friends and family for months

2= anger and resentment for years

1= unable or unwillingness of letting go of anger and resentment

■ Forgiveness

5= easily forgive enemies

4= easily forgive family and friends

3= never forgive enemies

2= never forgive friends or family

1= never forgive and refuse to speak about it

■ Creativity/learning (people in education or profession of life-long
learning qualify for a five)

5= sixty minutes or more five days per week

4= twenty to thirty minutes five days per week of hobby craft
or mind exercise like chess

3= occasionally

2= rarely

1= never

- **Depression/sadness/loneliness**
  5= rarely
  4= annually or seasonally
  3= most of the time
  2= controlled with medication
  1= uncontrolled with medication

- **Laughter/dance/sing**
  5= daily
  4= weekly
  3= annually
  2= rarely
  1= never

- **Vitamins/minerals and supplements**
  5= daily consumption
  4= weekly
  3= episodically
  2= occasionally
  1= rarely or never

- **Safety rules**
  5= follow rules to the letter
  4= most of the time
  3= only when required by law
  2= infrequently follow rules
  1= never follow rules (example helmet wearing)

- **Occupation/school/career**
  5= very low risk or semi-retired
  4= retired
  3= moderate risk
  2= high risk
  1= very high risk (example, police officer)

■ Volunteer work or charity

5= daily

4= weekly

3= monthly or seasonally

2= only when asked

1= rarely

■ Criminal/drug or alcohol history

5= no history

4= occasions of drug and alcohol excess

3= regular use of recreational drugs

2= daily use, including tabacco, vape or chew

1= daily use with an ongoing criminal history

■ Spiritual foundation/environment

5= rural living with daily routine

4= large inner city dwelling and a daily routine

3= country living with a seasonal spiritual routine

2= little to no spiritual foundation but open to explore new ideas

1= no belief system and closed minded to new idea (rural living is believed to be less stressful than urban)

■ Travel or Commute - any form (increase risk of injury)

5= very little

4= seasonally

3= monthly for work or pleasure

2= weekly commute

1= daily subway commute or weekly cross country travel or routine intercontinental travel.

This test is subjective, and you may not have all the exact information you need as you answer some of the questions posed. You may also disagree with the ratings and importance attributed to various parameters in each question. Be that as it may, several years back while in prison, a gay elderly priest took this test and scored an eighty-three, which has been the best score so far. He liked the concept and was able to reflect on areas of self enhancement. Obviously your experience may differ, and I think those with the lowest scores have the most to gain from this guide.

Maliks Holistic Spoke Wheel

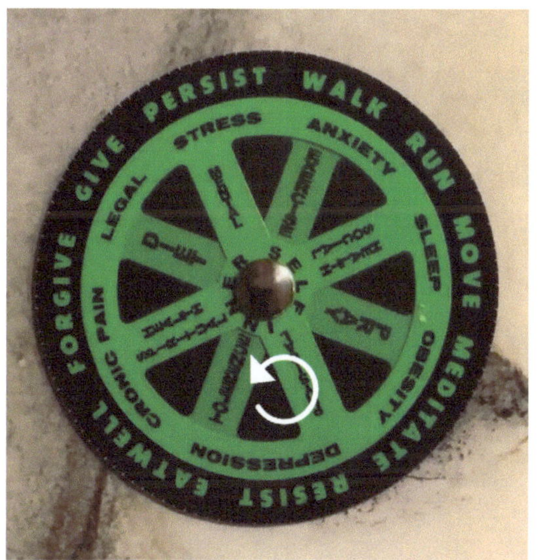

Medical innovation and technology have led to miraculous outcomes at a valuable price. The downplaying of prevention by the medical community and the public in general has made it more important to get back to the basics. The bulk of medical literature and the bombardment of conflicting scientific information can be confusing and discouraging to begin the important work of a daily and personalized prevention program. I take a holistic approach to fighting disease and preventing illness. I created a schematic diagram below to better explain Malik's holistic spoke wheels. It is used to gain a better understanding of what is important to prevent disease, stay well, and hopefully advance longevity.

Malik's Holistic Spoke Wheel

The human body has the tremendous capacity to heal itself through cell division and cellular repair, but first we must learn to listen to our body because it will tell us what it needs and when it needs it.

PHYSICAL HEALTH can be divided into four areas to consider:

1. Cardiovascular health, which is essentially the condition of your blood vessels and heart, can be monitored by checking your blood pressure and heart rate both at rest and with exercise. Normal blood pressure varies between 90/60 mmhg and 160/90 mmhg. Heart rate varies between 60 and 100 bpm. The lower the blood pressure and heart rate, generally speaking, the lower the risk for disease, as long as there are no symptoms or other reasons like adverse effects of drugs or infection that lead to sepsis and cardiovascular shock.

2. Endocrine/metabolism. This area includes obesity, diabetes mellitus, and lipids. Obesity is a big concern for many Americans and is linked to hypertension, heart disease, diabetes, degenerative joint disease, and certain cancers. It contributes to depression and a general lack of wellness. The most effective and lasting ways to stay the appropriate weight is calorie control. Currently the best method to determine the amount of fat in your body is by checking your BMI, body mass index. It should be less than twenty. It is based on a weight divided by height formula. You can use a less accurate "rule of five" method, which is 100 pounds for the first five feet and five pounds for every inch thereafter, give or take 5 percent. If you are five-foot five—inches tall then your appropriate weight should be 125 to 135 pounds. This would closely correlate with less the 20 percent BMI. Another important number is your cholesterol. Your body produces 60 percent of the cholesterol it uses because it is an important precursor to many hormones and transport molecules that your body needs to function. Cholesterol molecules are complex and are divided into good and bad, HDL and LDL respectively. Triglycerides (TG) is also part of the fat and lipids profile. Forming triglycerides is how your body stores calories. Total cholesterol should be less than 200 mg/dl with HDL more than 35 and LDL less than 100. TG should be about 100 to 150 mg/dl. Some people have a genetic predisposition to develop lipid abnormalities. For most of us, it is our dietary habits that worsen our lipid profile. Adult onset or type 2 diabetes go hand in hand with obesity, especially in North America, while type 1 or juvenile onset diabetes is genetic in origin. Diabetes, hypertension, hyperlipidemia, and obesity are all risk factors for heart attack and stroke primarily because of damage to blood vessels. Normal sugar or glucose level should be between 60 and 100 mg/dl. Normal glycohemoglobin or HgA1C is less than 5.5. Well-controlled diabetes comes with a glycohemoglobin less than 6.5

3. Immune system/inflammation. Doctors are beginning to understand the relationship between inflammation and disease. Inflammation affects the joints and connective tissues. Connective tissue is made from specialized cells and is practically everywhere in the body. It encases all the vital organs, as well as all blood vessels and lymphatic system. Many things can cause or aggravate inflammation, including infections and diet. For example viral infections can lead to inflammation of cardiac muscle and result in cardiomyopathy. The stronger your immune system is, the less likely there will be inflammation in the body. It appears that a balance of rest and exercise, as well as vitamin C, seem to help boost the immune system. In medicine we use many anti-inflammation drugs. They work but have a lot of side effects. There are numerous claims that certain herbal remedies help, but it appears that preventing the weakening of immunity is the key. For example we know that smoking cigarettes can lower immunity. Inflammation plays an important role in mediating heart disease and cancer, as well as other diseases. Currently there are inflammation markers that can be detected by blood. Sedimentation rate, CRP, and BNP are some blood tests that can be elevated when there is inflammation. It is well-established that gingival infection and inflammation can lead to heart disease, as well as blood vessels and joints. Inflammation in the body causes symptoms like pain and malaise. As with most medical issues, an ounce of prevention is worth a pound of cure. It starts with proper diet, exercise, and oral and skin hygiene.

4. Genetic factors and other considerations. The study of genetics and the relatively new field of epigenetics will have a tremendous impact on treatment of disease that have long affected man. A genetic affliction can have a significant impact on longevity and quality of life. Genetic diseases, like cystic fibrosis, muscular dystrophy, and Huntington's chorea, will one day have meaningful treatment and even a cure. It appears that we have genetic peculiarities that do not manifest as disease unless or until it is triggered by some mechanisms in the body. This may explain why some smokers don't get lung cancer and other who never smoke get lung cancer. Also, we used to think that there is nothing that can be done about your genes, and that may be true to a certain extent, but we know that our behaviors are passed down from generations and can be eventually encoded in our DNA. Heart disease, diabetes, obesity, certain cancers, and mental illness seem to run in my family and trying to maintain a balance and a homeostasis, although difficult would create long-term wellness and longevity.

One of my biggest struggles has been using marijuana to treat my ailments from childhood post-traumatic stress and depression to work related hepatitis C and its toxic treatment with interferon injections. It left me with arthralgia (joint pain) and fibromyalgia (muscle pain), as well as worsening my depression. I say biggest struggle because of the unique position I was in as a doctor using an illegal substance for years as a medication for himself and recommending it for my patients, all the while hiding it from family and friends whose beliefs were different, only for it to become legalized by the government and approved by the medical community. In 2003 I got a misdemeanor charge for possession of small amount of marijuana for personal use in Michigan. Marijuana was not legal at the time, and this led to some of my legal and employment issues, as I was ostracized by the medical community and began working as a vagabond or freelance physician in multiple settings. This worsened my mental health, as I was dealing with my father's death and starting a new practice in my home state. I enrolled in the HPRP (health professional recovery program) to protect my licensure and to get better. I completed HPRP in 2008. In 2009 marijuana was legalized in my home state. That same year, I had my second shoulder operation. The stress began to take a toll on my mental health.

MENTAL HEALTH can be divided into four areas to consider:

1. Cognition. This is essentially how smart you are and your ability to solve simple and complex problems, but I also think that this includes more importantly your curiosity level. The ability to focus and concentrate for certain periods of time and the ability to perform and complete various tasks. Our cognitive ability sets us apart from all other known life and indeed other primates. We have 200 to 300 billion cells that form our brain and nervous system that we are born with and must cultivate over a twenty-five-year period, from learning to walk and read, to developing our higher cortical centers for executive function. The neurons are protected by a myelin sheath, and these cells, neurons, communicate through synapses, and like all human cells, have a bilipid cell membrane to communicate with one another. It appears that a diet rich in omega fish oil helps with conduction of neurons and cell communication in general.

2. Memory. One of the most devastating illnesses of recent times and affects millions is Alzheimer's dementia. Dementia in general is caused by deterioration in mental capacity and the degeneration the neurons and synapses. It is associated with depression and rapidly declining physical health. Research is underway to determine the cause and find useful treatment. However, most causes of dementia are cerebrovascular or metabolic or toxic and can be prevented. Humans vary in their capacity to memorize as an exercise. Memory including recent, remote, cellular, and muscle memory are ways an organism uses its ability to survive and indeed thrive in its environment. Humans are similar. Yet we differ in that we can make choices and perform routine exercises to sharpen and strengthen our mental capacity.

3. Sleep. Sleep and memory seem to be physiologically and metaphysically linked. We often have to write down our dreams almost immediately if we want to remember them. Dreams are sometimes related to the memories of the wake world. People have different capacities for dreaming and remembering their dream or even controlling what they dream about. Dreams are as mysterious as sleep itself. One thing for certain is all organisms need sleep, seemingly to restore energy to continue living. We humans need six to ten hours of sleep nightly. Some can get by on four or five, but that's usually not sustainable. Sleep is probably one of the most studied but least understood of the many complicated body functions. Sleep is cyclical and rhythmic, and it is divided into stages with REM (rapid eye movement) being important and where we get our most restful sleep. Insomnia is one of the world's most common, non-life threatening ailments and is usually a symptom of an underlying issue like depression or anxiety. Work-related sleep deprivation and shift-related insomnia is a pandemic in itself and can lead to serious accidents and general deterioration of health. It is never a good idea to use alcohol or drugs to sleep because of side effects, addiction, and even unintentional death (think Michael Jackson). What seems to help is a healthy exercise routine, meditation, and being able to listen to your body because it will tell you when to sleep. Some cultures believe that taking a short nap at midday, like the Mexican siesta, is healthy for the mind, body, and soul.

4. Genetic and other consideration. Some people are prone to develop mental illness because it runs in their family, like schizophrenia or bipolar disease. There are various degrees of mental illness, and an individual can adapt and be highly functioning. For example you would want to have a neurosurgeon who is somewhat obsessive/compulsive about surgical details on your team, an individual who suffers from OCD will typically pay close attention to detail and time. There is much we don't understand about the genetics of mental illness, but the environment seems to play an important role in the severity of illness and the degree of response to treatment. Society has gotten much better at how it treats the disenfranchised members of its classes, but unfortunately many of them are homeless, mentally ill, and are no longer connected with their families. Finally, when we struggle with mental illness, our physical and spiritual health deteriorates, and visa-versa. So there is a way to practice mental hygiene daily as you would physical hygiene; for example avoiding cigarette smoke is beneficial physically. From a mental health perspective, it gives you control, confidence, and eventually better sleep. Quitting may also help foster healthy relationships. Mental and spiritual hygiene could include the choice to stop using foul language or indiscriminately watching porn. While porn and foul language are not inherently wrong, it could be seen as unclean in terms of mental and spiritual hygiene that goes against the grain of the development of your authentic self.

SOCIAL HEALTH

1. Relationships. It is a long-held belief that long-standing healthy relationships, like marriage, leads to longevity and improved quality of life. Children depend on their parents to get through life, and grandparents depend on their children to usher them in their old age as the grandparents' abilities fade. Relationships are based on trust, honesty, and the value we place on one another's friendship. Many problems arise from unhealthy relationships, including abuse, depression, anxiety, adultery, illegal activities, addiction, and even death. It is important to understand that the two most fundamental positions in resolving an argument is that both parties respect each other's space and offer the other the chance to communicate his or her side. Relationships extend beyond marriage and into our workplace. By maintaining an open mind and having a clear sense of your values, you can set priorities and create appropriate balance in your relationships. Sometimes we have unresolved relationships with persons who have since died, and the only way to get past it may only come through professional help. It is clear that bad relationships lead to bad emotions. The word *emotion* means energy in motion. Emotions are the response to feelings generated by circumstance or a source. It is now believed that negative human emotions, such as anger and resentment, can lead to physical disease. Our thoughts lead to our action and eventually becomes energy that escapes into the human world for consumption; if the energy is negative, it will carry negative karma, and if positive, then it will have a positive message that can be shared. Karma in Hindu and eastern philosophy is believed to be the sum of all of your actions in this and previous existence. I feel that our life's memories are stored in our brain cells (DNA) as a form of energy that periodically affect our emotions. I think that a good deal of this energy is carried with us in the afterlife as a form of tangible memories that connect us all to a higher consciousness. Think of a time where a thought or a memory of a long-deceased loved one comes to mind and with it an emotion. The best way to manage relationships is to have the inner gift of forgiveness and be in a relatively consistent state of gratitude.

2. Community service. This is an important part of your social health. It keeps you connected. It gives your life value and provides confidence to move forward. It is especially rewarding if you find joy in helping other. Community service begins in childhood when children learn to share and continues on to old age. People always tell me the they feel best when they give. Giving has many definitions, and it is important to give out of charity rather than out of obligation. Giving from the heart means that when you give out of charity, this helps open your seventh chakra by operating through the pineal gland in the brain, which releases energy. Our third chakra is our heart and is naturally magnetic, which means that it draws energy in and thus the sometimes overwhelming joy that we see in giving.

3. Work/school/career/hobbies. You career choice is based on your skills, likes and dislikes, physical and mental abilities, and some-times location. If based solely on income, it will not be long-lasting or ful-filling. I always tell anyone who asks about career choices that their path should be something that brings joy. Do you laugh or sing at your work-place, and do you look forward to working or doing whatever it is daily? Remember, going to the best school or having the highest paying job will not bring you happiness.

4. Legal consideration. This is taking into account living a re-sponsible life from literally not jay walking to having a trusted lawyer re-view contracts and assist with all legal matters. The stress of illegal behavior is physically and mentally harmful, not to mention the guns, drugs, and violence that comes with criminal activity. I am definitely not a saint, and I began jaywalking at a young age, but as a successful physician using marijuana illegally and hiding it from everyone, including my wife and patients, became too much of a strain. I am sure it affected my blood pressure and anxiety level. Unfortunately, in today's society, it appears that some people get into more legal trouble than others, either because of per-sonality or color or class difference. Social justice does indeed swing on a pendulum and occasionally shifts in favor of the disenfranchised. Individ-ually we can help each other by respecting the law and allowing honest and fair policies to create a peaceful work and school environment.

SPIRITUAL HEALTH

1. Inner self. This is the faith inside you that drives you to wake up daily and look forward to what may come. It provides a sense of belonging to a much larger source of energy and that somewhere in this or another dimension, there is an eternity to our being (a reason for our being in this space and at this time). It is the reason for our being.

2. Outer self. This is that part of you where hope and confidence come together and allow your physical appearance to shine. It is all of the abilities you use to connect with your environment on an individual level or as a group. It is the movement or the transfer of energy between people in the same sphere. This is where confidence in yourself is developed, how you show yourself to the rest of the world. Or put another way how you view yourself. From purely a psychological stand, this would be the area of the ego and super ego, where you develop a sense of who you are and how the world perceives you.

3. Acceptance. This is an area where many of us reach a sticking point in our lives. Acceptance is the willingness to realize your station in life and understand that it is a dynamic process. All things are subject to change. It is taking responsibility for any decisions you make and paying the consequences for the actions you take. It is also accepting the conditions of your surroundings and being at peace with it while moving forward. It is healthy not to accept certain things as a way to motivate or create an avenue for change, and sometimes it is difficult to know if change is needed. A close and similar approach is the concept of tolerance. A key to cellular and an organism's survival is tolerance to its environment. Tolerance is a form of acceptance, tolerating one another.

4. Forgiveness. Many of us struggle with anger, I know I do. Many of us hold on to that anger with negative self-talk. We all have self-talk. Self-talk is what you go around telling yourself all day. It's usually reminding yourself of things or events revolving around work, family, or yourself. When you find yourself blaming yourself or others for things that anger, upset, or frustrate, try to forgive both yourself and the other without judging one way or the other. Think of this as negative energy that you are releasing. Negative energy can cause physical and mental harm. This is difficult to do gracefully and is dependent on the severity of the issue. A case that comes to mind is a man who actually went to the prison where his son's murderer was incarcerated and physically met with him and forgave him. This unleashed an energy and a spirit from both of them that brought the father peace, the murderer partial redemption, and hopefully eternal rest for the deceased. I'm sure this was not easy to do, but there must have been something in forgiving that allowed him to let go, and that created a pathway for healing. That's the level of healing that some gurus feel occurs involving the seventh chakra. This is a deep subject, and many philosophers have written on it. One of the most popular and oldest prayers (The Lord's prayer, Holy Bible, Matthew 6:9-13) is given to us by Jesus says "…forgive us our trespasses as we forgive those who trespass against us…"

DIET

1. Carbohydrates are the biggest source of immediate energy for your nourishment. They provide 4 cal/gm. All carbohydrates and indeed all food is eventually broken down to glucose that is used to make energy at the cellular level. Glucose is the simplest form of sugar. Many fruits are simple carbohydrates. Carbohydrates are either simple, complex, or mixed (ie. vegetables, seeds, and grains and are known as starches). Carbohydrates should be about 30 percent of your daily nourishment. Fiber is important in digestive health and may improve lipid profile, as well as prevent certain cancers. About thirty grams per day is needed, and the only way to get it is by eating mixed and complex carbohydrates, like oatmeal.

2. Proteins are the building blocks of every cell and are required for cell function and repair to energy production and muscle building. Proteins are needed for immunity and reproduction. The healthiest source of protein for meat eaters is fish, eggs, and soy for vegetarians. Other sources of protein include all meats, whey, legumes, tree nuts, seeds, grains, beans, and rice. Thirty percent of your diet should be protein. Some people eat a diet rich in protein or take protein supplements to help build muscle and as an initial weight loss regimen, such as the Atkins diet. Too much protein, however, is hard on the kidneys and the digestive track. Proteins also provide 4 cal/gm.

3. Fats provide the greatest source of energy at nine calories per gram. It is impossible to avoid all fats in the diet. Fats are needed for energy storage, transport of molecules across cellular membranes important for cellular communication at every single cell in the body. That's what makes consuming fish oil important in longevity and brain function. It also helps with joint mobility. There are two kind of fats, saturated and unsaturated. Unsaturated are better for your health and are liquid at room temperature, like olive oil and vegetable oil. Lard and butter are solid at room temperature and are less healthy. Fats should be between 20 and 30 percent of your diet depending on your needs. A growing teenager would require 30 percent, and an adult trying to lose weight and lower the risk of heart disease should limit fats to 20 percent and avoid saturated fats altogether.

4. Other considerations including liquid intake. Liquids, specifically water, is extremely important for digestion and cellular function.

Adequate amount of clean water daily is recommended with limiting coffee, tea, and alcohol while avoiding or restricting sugary drinks, like soda pop or Kool-Aid. Fresh fruits and vegetables contain a lot of water. Currently the most recommended diet is the zone diet, which is 30 percent fat, 30 percent carbohydrates, and 30 percent protein. Historically the healthiest diet is the Mediterranean diet, which is rich in green leafy vegetables, olive oil, grains, and nuts, as well as middle eastern and oriental spices that provide additional health benefits. Also, the Okinawa diet is excellent and is based on Japanese cuisine rich in seafood and raw veggies and smaller frequent portions rather than three large meals daily. Our body expends 750 to 1,000 calories daily for basic metabolic function, such as brain function and energy production and storage. Most of us require about 2,000 to 3,500 calories per day to go about our routine daily task. Someone, like an active sumo wrestler, may require up to five or 6,000 calories daily. The point being what we don't use gets stored as fat. The word *sugar* has many meanings, but in medical terms it refers to glucose. One of the main functions of the body is to produce glucose and pump it, along with oxygen, through the cardiovascular system to the brain for 24/7 consumption. Having a healthy heart and eating the right foods will keep your brain healthy. Regular and ritualistic fasting have physical and spiritual benefits. I hate saying this because I know how popular alcohol is, and I occasionally like a glass of red wine, cold beer, or good scotch, but another reason alcohol consumption may be harmful is it gives seven calories per gram of "empty calories," which means no nutritional value. Chronic use can deplete your body of some vitamins, like B12 and folate. It can cause liver toxicity and failure not to mention the hundred other things that alcoholism causes, from depression to dementia. When I was younger, I and many of my compadres believed a myth that you could work off the negative effects of alcohol by vigorous exercise. This is not true.

EXERCISE

1. Aerobic exercise is the best for the cardiovascular system. It includes walking, running, swimming, hiking, biking, yoga, kayaking, basketball, baseball, soccer, gymnastics, and so much more.

2. Anaerobic means without oxygen. Simply put it means your cells are metabolizing with lower levels of oxygen for the amount of work that the muscle cells are doing. Anaerobic exercise is important for muscle strength and building. The best example is weight-lifting, and a byproduct of this anaerobic process is lactic acid. Lactic acidosis forms crystals and builds up along the muscle strands and is one of the reasons muscles become sore the next day.

3. Stretching is vital to muscle health and connective tissues. We have muscle everywhere, including our digestive track and the miles of smooth muscle lining our arteries, veins, and lymphatic system throughout our body. There are different types of stretching exercises. It is important to involve all the joints in the body throughout the day and spend about ten minutes or more stretching the major muscle groups. Cool down and warm up stretching exercise prevent muscle and joint injury.

4. Breathing sounds simple, but we spend a lot of time subconsciously holding our breath. You are probably holding your breath now. Our brain controls our breathing spontaneously in the respiratory center where minute detection in carbon dioxide levels control the diaphragm, which is the largest respiratory muscle. It separates the abdomen from the chest and will contract voluntarily or involuntarily, depending on the body needs. We can live without food a couple weeks and without water a couple days, but only fifteen to thirty minutes without oxygen. Respirations are about five to twenty-five breaths per minute depending on whether we are sleeping or exercising. Breathing exercises become very important in meditation. We tend to hold our breath under stressful situations. The most important thing you can do is to take a deep breath and learn to regulate your breathing. Once mastered breathing techniques can instantaneously release an energy and provide calming and soothing feelings where tension was causing malaise. I do this frequently with meditation to get instant drop in my blood pressure and to relieve headaches and neck tension.

MEDITATION

1. Stress reduction and pain control. The breathing exercise in meditation almost immediately creates a reduction in stress by controlling the amount of neurotransmitter being discharged. In fact, through hypnosis and meditation, people have been able to tolerate the pain of surgery with minimal anesthesia, and in some cases, no anesthesia at all.

2. Energy restoration. The process of meditation allows for your cells to rest while you focus on the mind. There are specific mindful meditations exercise that you can do, and with practice, become proficient at redirecting energy flow in your body, which may provide for specific or targeted healing. For example heart palpitations, anxiety, headaches, or nausea can sometimes be treated this way.

3. Realignment or opening chakras. Eastern medicine has been around and helping people for seven thousand years and teaches us that the body has seven areas, where movement of energy occurs in relation to body function. The nerves innervating these areas are facilitated through the brain and spinal column. It is believed that energy may become trapped in some areas and can cause symptoms or disease states. Some obvious examples include anger that raises blood pressure and causes a heart attack or stroke. The developing back pain as a result of improper diet and constipation. The lowers chakras involve digestive and reproductive processes and is what connects you with Mother Nature. It connects you to your ancestral origins and Earth. The higher chakras have to do with cardiovascular and respiratory centers, as well as the head and neck, which control communication and emotions, and connects you with your environment. It takes a special skill to reach or open the seventh chakra, which is the highest, and aligns you with the cosmos and your higher power or the collective conscience.

4. Practice daily meditation from a few minutes several times daily. Try different methods, like breathing in and out while repeating a simple mantra or imaginary relaxation at the beach focusing on waves while feeling the warmth of the sun on your shoulder. Another good meditation is a type of mindfulness and is to focus inward to the desired body parts while breathing in and out and concentrating on healing energy flowing through the blood vessels and lymphatics, allowing the power of the

body to heal itself. With practice a person can meditate practically any-
where and anytime, and in fact some monks will meditate for hours. Meditation and prayer are not the same, but many people do them together. In
fact meditation is using the brain and mind toward healing the body by tun-
ing down certain central nervous system neurotransmitters, allowing for
relaxation or amplifying others to soothe chronic pain or headache.

PRAYER

1. Prayer is about the non-self, whereas meditation is about the self. When we pray, we use uniquely human attributes that allow for connection with a higher power, being, source, creator, collective consciousness, Mother Nature, the sun, the universe, the big mystery, Allah, or God. Prayer is probably the oldest form of medical therapy and oftentimes is used as last hope for the severely ill and dying. Even though prayer is about the non-self, I think the phrase heal thyself mean to also pray for yourself, for your health, and even for your salvation or the salvation of others. Dharma is the relationships you have with your higher power. Karma is the energy that flows through that relationship and since we are all connected to a higher conciseness, so our karma is connected to each of us.

2. Inner voice. This is the voice inside you that controls your self-talk when it becomes irrational. Irrational self-talk is not based on objective fact and is not based in reality. It results in bringing harm to the self and relationships. The self-talk is the mind reacting to its emotions, and the inner voice is above it and works at the level of the seventh chakra, or what is sometimes called the third eye. The anatomical location in the brain is the pineal gland and certain hormones are secreted that control body functions and regulate the twenty-four hour circadian rhythm. Prayer is a spiritual energy that flows as it does in the trillions of cells on the human body. It becomes no surprise that prayer provides for many explained and unexplained miracles that have occurred in medical and religious communities throughout our short history on this earth.

3. Relieve suffering. The Quran says and the Bible suggests that we are born into hardship and that suffering is brought onto man as punishment for original sin, and redemption comes only with grace. Grace is given to us and cannot be earned nor bought. When we suffer, we are experiencing a negative energy somewhere in our body and with prayer and meditation you have an avenue to partially relieve discomfort at the body level and alleviate tension at the mental and even the spiritual level. In this area, prayer should be looked at as using the energy of an optimistic outlook to give thanks for the many gifts we are afforded. My wife says that God is always giving us gifts, but we rarely recognize it, or don't want it, because the gift is usually wrapped in crappy wrapping paper. What that means is that we don't want to open the gifts because they don't look appealing to us when it is exactly the thing we need. Prayer is often used by a community to relieve discord at the social level.

4. Gratitude is a key to relieve stress and suffering by simple energy flow. We search for a constant state of happiness because this allows us to mask, hide, or ignore our pain and suffering. This search itself causes pain and anxiety through addiction, mental illness, and relationships issues, as well as through legal troubles. By having unconditional gratitude for your circumstance and allowing the process of "…letting go and letting God…" to expel all negative energy or emotions. This practice changes the search from constant happiness (which is unsustainable or unachievable) and dissolve into a state of infinite joy. Every time you decide to let go and breath in and allow yourself to let happen whatever will happen, releasing all the negative emotions or energies that come with holding on, you can really appreciate the sense of infinite joy and peace that come with that decision.

EXAMPLE OF A MEDITATION/PRAYER

The house in the meadow (HIM) meditation.

This is a type of imagery meditation that I some time use for both my body healing, as well as prayer for my spiritual fulfillment.

Imagine yourself walking on partially shaded trail adjacent to a field of tall grass on a warm sunny day. The rays of the sun soothe your shoulders as you brush your finger tips on the tall silky grass, inhaling the faint aroma of flowers in the meadow. As you are imagining this, relax all of the muscles in your body beginning with your feet and toes and work your way up to your legs, then back, neck, and shoulders. Relax all of your facial muscles in your forehead, jaws, and eyes. As you do this, concentrate on the level of the spinal column which innervates these muscles. Slowly breathing in and exhaling out as you let go of all negative feelings and emotions.

As you are lazily and effortlessly strolling, the path curves into a meadow where it gives to a beautiful welcoming grove of trees shading an area that has been set for you to sit and be welcomed with food of your choice by an elderly lady who is familiar with you. She welcomes you and guides through the grove to the other side where the meadow continues with even more dazzling flowers. You continue feeling the warmth of the sun. As it begins to slowly set as you approach the most elegant yet simple cabin with a comfortable porch swing, rocking chairs, a small table with prepared freshly-squeezed lemonade, and a figure sitting in one of the chairs. Continue breathing and relaxing your muscles.

This figure is, for me, Jesus. It can be Mohammad, Buddha, your deceased grandparent, anyone that you trust, or even the mirror image of yourself. This person knows you so well that with a simple hug and no spoken words, you are able to convey all of your worries and desires and be met with a grace that can only be offered through this person. You are invited to sit and stay as long as you want, and if tired, you may enter and nap in a room that is arranged just for your comfort. You give thanks for the moment and everything that comes with it without any conditions on yourself or others. At this point you may pray for healing for yourself and/or others.

And when you are ready to return the same way you came, knowing that the house in the meadow is always there for your return.

In conclusion this approach helped me try to prioritize from a health and wellness standpoint what is important and to mute out all the additional and sometimes unnecessary information we get from those who try to help us, including the medical community. The holistic wheel is not perfect but does allow for improvement in your life. I have also included some daily suggestions that really bring together some key points to remind you of what's important, stay well, and prevent disease and hopefully live longer and healthier.

25 of MALIK'S MEDICAL PEARLS

1. Adequate hydration
2. Avoid excess (gambling, shopping, eating…etc)
3. Avoid risky behavior (unprotected sex or motorbike without helmet)
4. Balance diet
5. Balance work, rest, play time
6. Follow the Golden Rule. Treat others as you would yourself.
7. Regular fasting
8. Foster healthy relationships and limit unhealthy ones
9. Total body hygiene, including teeth
10. Mental and spiritual hygiene
11. Immunize when you can
12. Follow all safety rules
13. Low dose aspirin if not contraindicated, for prevention and treatment of heart attack, stroke, and thrombosis
14. Multivitamin with iron for women. Add calcium if over 50 and B-complex if consuming alcohol regularly
15. Multivitamin without iron for men and B-complex if consuming alcohol regularly (and yes, beer is alcohol)
16. Limit diet to healthy fats, like olive oil or nuts
17. Limit protein source to mostly fish, eggs, soybean, baked chicken, and unprocessed meats
18. Eat a diet rich and varied in cruciferous and green leafy vegetables and fruits like berries, melons, and apples
19. Omega fish oil daily, unless allergic.
20. Vitamin C 500 or more daily. 2000 mg when ill with viral infaction.
21. Annual health and wellness exams
22. Read at least ten to fifteen minutes daily.
23. Develop a daily ritual or mantra that you tell yourself, like, "I will live today like it's my last, or I will be kind to others, or I will enjoy what comes my way."
24. Laugh and dance frequently
25. Cry periodically and appropriately like at funerals or when feeling particularly sad.

I was feeling particularly sad one cold, February day and was crying uncontrollably. After twenty months at McKean Federal Prison, I was transferred to another prison. For logistical and security reasons, I was not notified and neither was my family. And the way the feds do things, what could have been a short distance bus trip turned out to be a three-week, shackled, 2,000-mile partial bus and federal airplane ride with armed marshals spent mostly in twenty-three-hour solitary confinement until I reached my final destination.

I was denied a transfer furlough, and I was upset that they had also denied me several furloughs in the past. When my brother, Majed, got severely ill and eventually died, I tried desperately for three weeks to get an emergency furlough even for twenty-four hours to be with him, and I was denied for no apparent reason. A large factor in my agreeing to not try the case and accept a plea is I was advised that I would serve my time in a federal camp, and it was easy, and I would be given furlough and even conjugal visits with my wife. What a lie that turned out to be. I was in solitary confinement and crying when I began to feel an empathy for that eight-year-old boy who felt anxious and angry as a child and now as an adult. I also began to feel an empathy for all of those suffering from mental illness and addiction and all of the victims and their families. My empathy led to a gratitude that began quietly inside me that to this day, I begin all of my prayers with gratitude.

Human happiness and prosperity throughout the ages have been primarily guided by two opposing principles: love and hate. They are also know by many other names, such as trust and deceit, truth and lies, good and evil, friend and foe, give and receive, create and destroy, peace and war, faith and fear, and more. We are fortunately on the same journey with similar physical and psychological struggles and want good tidings for ourselves and loved ones.

Many patients don't realize that a doctor begins his examination with the handshake and a glance at the biggest organ in the human body: the integumentary system, AKA the skin. It usually provides the first clues to illness or nutritional status, for example, pallor points to anemia and lack of iron. Jaundice or yellowing refers to liver ailments, or uremia (bronze color) denotes kidney disease. Cachexia or wasting is caused by cancer or malnutrition and mental illness. There is so much more like rashes and bruising and the evidence that these clues point to.

We live in an increasingly fast-paced and ever-changing world, and it is important to slow down and take frequent self-assessment of yourself and your environment. Obviously your age and station in life will determine that and some you will be forced to take a closer look by the medical or legal community.

I recommend these guidelines for anyone who wants to get healthy and to use balance as an approach to achieve wellness and longevity. **It is my desire to empower people to take charge.**

Acknowledgements

I wish to thank the many patients, friends, and family that let me be part of their lives and allowed me to care for them and learn from them. I also want to thank the many instructors, colleagues, students, and mentors who by their willingness to teach and learn were instrumental in advancing a holistic approach to wellness and disease prevention. I also want to thank my parents and siblings for their unwavering support.

Lastly I want to thank my wife and best friend, Avelina, who encouraged me to go to medical school. She has been my true colleague, and for this, my sounding board and one person who can critique me as objectively as well. I have never met a more ethical doctor. I indeed wonder why she has stayed with me, but indeed she has through thick and thin. I want to give special thanks to my children Amir, Leighla, Yazmin, and Aleena for their love and patience.

I would be remiss not to mention the countless number of people, including healthcare providers, researchers, spiritual leaders, teachers, healers, friends, and family, who have acted as my mentors and through their companionship. I gained a higher level of love and understanding that to this day carries me forward to a better understanding of healing from a holistic viewpoint, and you know who you are.